ERECTILE DYSFUNCTION: Treat And Prevent ED Permanently!

The Secrets Herbs & Steps To Cure: Male Impotence, Premature Ejaculation, Low Perm Count, Swing Mood, Fatigue & How To Increased Sexual Urge (Libido) To Get & Keep Harder & Long Lasting Erection!

CLEMENT JACOB

Copyright Notice. By Clement Jacob

All rights reserved. No part of this book may be reproduced, copied or transmitted into any form or by any means, electronic or mechanical, including photocopy, recording or by any information, storage and retrieval system, without the written permission from the copyright owner.

Table of Contents

ERECTILE DYSFUNCTION: Treat And Prevent ED Permanently! 1

Introduction 7

CHAPTER ONE 9

   Review of Erection 9

      What Is An Erection? 9

      How Erection Takes Place/Happens? 10

      Types Of Erections? 12

      What Are The Component Of Male Sexual Functions? 14

CHAPTER TWO 15

   Review Of Erectile Dysfunction 15

      What Is Erectile Dysfunctions? 15

      What Are The Causes Of Erectile Dysfunction? .. 17

      What Are The Physiological Causes Of ED? 17

      What Are The Psychological Causes Of ED? 21

What Are The Physical Causes Of Erectile Dysfunction? 22

The Symptoms Or Signs Of Erectile Dysfunctions 25

CHAPTER THREE 26

Treat And Prevent ED Permanently.........................26

What Are the Needed Herbs for the Treatment Of erectile Dysfunctions?..26

Maca Root..26

Precaution And Side Effects Of Consuming Maca Root? 27

Maca Root Dosage 28

The Preparation of Maca Root 29

Ginkgo Biloba 30

Precaution and Side Effects of Consuming Ginkgo Biloba 31

Ginkgo Biloba Dosage 31

The Preparation of Ginkgo Biloba: 32

Irish Sea Moss..33

The Precaution and Side Effects Of Consuming Irish Sea Moss..34

The Dosage Of Irish Sea Moss 34

Preparation of Irish Sea Moss................................35

Panax Ginseng 35

The Precautions and Side Effects of Consuming Panax Ginseng 36

Dosage of Panax Ginseng 37

The Preparation of Panax Ginseng........................38

Yohimbe 39

The Precautions and Side Effects of Consuming Yohimbe 39

The Dosage of Yohimbe 41

The Preparation Of Yohimbe 42

CHAPTER FOUR..43

The Natural Remedy To Screw Your Woman Like A

Porm Star! 43

Steps On How To Treat And Prevent ED Permanently 43

Fruits And Veggies That Helps To Enhance Blood Flow To The Penis 44

Steps on How To Takes Your Herbs and Fruit. 49

How To Make Herbal Tea With Yohimbe, Maca Root And Panax Ginseng Combine? 66

How to Stretch Penis (Penis Stretching Exercise)? 67

About The Book 69

Erectile Dysfunction: Treat And Prevent ED Permanently!

Introduction

This book is design for male adult (from the age of 18) who are finding it difficult to get and sustain erection, men with small penis that desire a bigger, longer, thicker and harder and long lasting erection, men from the age of 50 and above that are finding it difficult to get and sustain erection for sexual intercourse, men who have lost their self-esteem because they have stop being the men they use to be in the bedroom, men who are suffering from swing mood, low libido, premature ejaculation, low sperm count, lack enough energy and stamina to screw their woman like a porn star and anything that is related to erectile dysfunctions.

In this guide, the author will walk you through a 21 day program on how you will cleanse your entire body system, treat impotence, premature ejaculation, low sperm count, boost libido, increased energy and stamina level and sustain a long lasting erection with a bigger, thicker, harder and longer penis to screw your woman like never before.

You don't want to miss this?

Grab your copy now!

CHAPTER ONE
Review of Erection
What Is An Erection?

An erection is the process whereby a man's penis stands erect in order for him to make love or have sexual intercourse and easily penetrate his woman's vagina and ejaculate semen. Usually, erections take place in a healthy man when he is sexually aroused or sexually excited or stimulated. Sometimes, it happens when the man is touched sexually or if he sees a naked woman or girl live or her picture or thinks about having sex with someone. Sometimes, it occurs without thinking of sex or being touched when one wakes up or during the night and sometimes, it happens unexpectedly.

How Erection Takes Place/Happens?

The penis has a banana or sausage shape with a duct or tube known as the "urethra" that run through the penis. Both the semen and urine passes through the urethra to get out of the body. The urethra is made up of tissue known as "the corpus spongiosum penis" this is a Latin word known as "body of the penis"

The penis has tissue that are close to the upper surface area (two cylindrical tissues) known as: corpora cavernosa penis (caves) and the other one is known as "corpus cavernosum" all these tissues have lots of blood vessels known as "arteries" that carries the blood.

Let's look at how erections take place now. Whenever a guy or man is sexually aroused or stimulated, which might arise as a result of a sexual touch which could be masturbation or touched by an opposite sex (woman) in a sexually way or when he sees or watch sexual pictures or pornography or a naked woman. Immediately, the nerves in the arteries of the two cylindrical tissues in the penis will cause a chemical known as nitric oxide to be released into the arteries which will compel it to dilate and be filled with blood. Now, all the tissues will now be filled with blood and the penis will become longer, larger, thicker, stronger and harder. Finally, the tissue known as 'corpora cavernosa' will press against the blood vessels known as 'veins' that helps in carrying of blood out of the penis and a valve will pop up to stops the urine from entering the urethra. This is why, only semen flows along the urethra and very difficult to urinate during erection.

Erections does not happen only through the above reasons

as it can happen when one imagine he is having sex with someone or sees a naked person. In this type of situation, the man's brain sends a signal or message to the penis through the spinal cord and an erection will take place. The most important thing about the brain is the fact that it can stop erections even if you are touched in a sexual way.

Once you have an orgasm and ejaculation or you are not sexually arouse, your erections will come to an end and your penis will become small again. The time it will take for your erection to fall depends on the length and thickness of your penis.

Types Of Erections?

Basically, there are two types of erections known as:

1. Erections when sleeping or morning glory or wood:

erection when sleeping is also known as 'nocturnal penile tumescence' this is the type of erections that occurs by itself when you are sleeping and dreaming. This type of erection usually occurs when your bladder is filled with urine which will lead to the pressing of your penis tissues and thus leading to an erection.

2. Unexpected erections or sudden or surprise (spontaneous) erection: this type of erection is common with teenagers and sometimes adult do experience this type of erections. This type of erection is an involuntary and is normal type of erection that can happen anytime at anywhere.

What Are The Component Of Male Sexual Functions?

There are three (3) important components of male sexual functions which include:

1. Libido: this has to do with the desire or interest for sexual intercourse.

2. Erection: this has to do with the ability to have and keep erection for sexual intercourse.

3. Ejaculation: this is the last component that has to do with orgasm and releasing of semen.

CHAPTER TWO
Review Of Erectile Dysfunction
What Is Erectile Dysfunctions?

Erectile dysfunction also known as "ED or male impotence" is a situation where a man (from the age of puberty upward) finds it difficult to get and sustain an erection or to have or keep an erection of his penis for sexual intercourse. In other word, it is a type of sexual dysfunction whereby the penis fails to become or stay erect during sexual activity.

To achieve and sustain erections, the process is complex as it involved lots of organs known as:

1. The brain
2. The blood circulation
3. The hormones
4. The nerves

5. The blood

6. The muscle

7. The tissues

However, once there is any issue with any of the above or the malfunctions of any of the above, there will be erectile dysfunction. Erectile dysfunction does not have age as it can happen to anyone at any age but it's very common to age people.

Today, more than 50% of men from the age of 50 and above are suffering from mild form of erectile dysfunction which if it is not treated; might lead to complete erectile dysfunction. Furthermore, 5% of men from the age of 40 are suffering from complete erectile dysfunctions, 15% from the age of 70 upward.

What Are The Causes Of Erectile Dysfunction?

The causes of erectile dysfunctions can be categories into three which I name as the 3P's of erectile dysfunctions. These causes or P's include:

1. Physiological causes of ED
2. Psychological or environmental causes of ED
3. Physical or organic causes of ED

What Are The Physiological Causes Of ED?

The physiological causes of Ed have to do with any physiological problems that can affect your erection. Such problems include:

1. Problem with the brain or nervous system: any problem that can affect your brain and the nerves, can lead to erectile dysfunction. The common

problems or diseases that can affect the brain or nervous system include:

    i. Spinal cord and nerves problem

    ii. Alzheimer's disease

    iii. Parkinson's disease

    iv. Multiple sclerosis

    v. Stroke

    vi. Diabetes mellitus

    vii. Panic disorders

    viii. Schizophrenia

2. Circulatory problems: this type of problems has to do with any types of diseases that can affect the way your blood circulates in your whole body system. Such problems include:

i. Hypertension also known as 'high blood pressure' it occurs when the blood vessels are blocked which in turns will lead to less blood flowing into the penis.

ii. Smoking also reduces circulation as it causes the arteries to be too narrower. In fact, research have it that about 85% of people suffering with erectile dysfunctions are smokers

3. Hormonal problems: this type of problem has to do with any types of disease that can lead to the increase/decrease in the productions of sexual hormones. E.g.; diseases that affect the testicles or pituitary gland will certainly lead to erectile dysfunction. Some of this problems include:

i. Low testosterone

ii. Peyronie's disease

4. Problems that are caused by medical treatment and surgery: the damage of some of the nerves and blood vessels during surgery of prostate or rectum or bladder or colon (intestine) or some sort of medical treatment like; destroying of cancer cells through the use of radiation might lead to ED.

5. Some medications/drugs: some drugs or medications like: lithium that is administer to people that are suffering with bipolar can cause ED as it reduces the amount of nitric oxide in the blood vessels of the corpora cavernosa.

6. Lifestyle and age: your lifestyle determine whether you will suffer from ED early or not for instance,

people that consume too much alcohol and illegal drugs tend to suffer from ED very early in life and also, people that are old or obese tend to suffer from ED than skinny and younger men.

What Are The Psychological Causes Of ED?

The psychological causes of ED have to do with your psychological state of being. These causes include:

1. Lack of confidence: if you desire to have a sexual intercourse with someone that make you feel anxious or nervous, probably because you believe you are not in her league or you are not good at sex, you might end up having mild erectile dysfunction.

2. Poor communication with partner: If you are having issue with your partner that is affecting your

relationship which could lead to: arguments, fighting, facing a divorce, etc., you might experience some mild ED.

3. Stress/Depression: If you are feeling depress or stress due to big changes in your lifestyle, job or one thing or the other, there is high tendency of mild ED.

What Are The Physical Causes Of Erectile Dysfunction?

The physical causes of erectile dysfunction have to do with some physical reasons why people might suffer from erectile dysfunctions. These causes include:

1. Heart disease: once one has heart disease, his arteries will be affected and if the arteries are affected, he will suffer from shot flow of blood to the penis. Thereby making it difficult to sustain

erection.

2. Atherosclerosis: this lead to the narrowing or clogging of the blood vessels which in turns will lead to low blood flow into the penis making it impossible to sustain erection. However, if it is not treated, it might lead to heart attacks.

3. High cholesterol: this is another general cause of erectile dysfunctions as the higher the LDL level, the higher chances of erectile dysfunction. This is because, if you have high level of cholesterol, your body will find it difficult to produce the needed chemicals to sustain erection.

4. High blood pressure: (the same thing with circulation problem under physiological causes of Ed).

5. Diabetes: because diabetes, mostly type 2 diabetes have the potency to damage blood vessel and nerves which are very important for erections. If one is suffering from diabetes, he has a strong chance of suffering from erectile dysfunction if not treated.

6. Obesity: obesity on its own is an independent risk factor for erectile dysfunction.

7. Metabolic syndrome: this is another risk factor for erectile dysfunction that has to do with massive increased in blood pressure, high cholesterol, high insulin levels etc.

8. Sleep disorders: research has it that people with obstructive sleep apnea can affect testosterone and oxygen level which in turns can lead to erectile dysfunction.

The Symptoms Or Signs Of Erectile Dysfunctions

The symptoms and sign of erectile dysfunctions include:

1. Difficult to have erection

2. Difficult to keep an erection

3. Low libido or sexual urge

4. Low self-esteem or lack confidence

5. Feeling depressed

CHAPTER THREE
Treat And Prevent ED Permanently
What Are the Needed Herbs for the Treatment Of erectile Dysfunctions?

The needed herbs for the treatment of erectile dysfunctions include:

1. Maca root
2. Gingko Biloba
3. Irish Sea Moss
4. Panax Ginseng
5. Yohimbe

Maca Root

Maca root is a very effective herbal medicine that has been used by the Peruvians for over 3,000 years. This herb is very rich with some compound and nutrients like:

vitamins-B, fatty acids, amino acids, phytonutrients, zinc, calcium, selenium, magnesium and iron.

Till date this herb is very effective for the improvement of fertility (increase sperm count and semen) for men, enhance sexual urge (libido), treatment of erectile dysfunctions that is caused by antidepressants, anemia (tired blood), reliefs anxiety and depression, improve energy and stamina level, relief symptoms of menopause, boost the immune system etc.

Precaution And Side Effects Of Consuming Maca Root?

Till at the time of written this book, Maca root is 100% safe for men to consume except for women that it has some side effect which I am not going to talk about since this book is completely design for men.

Maca Root Dosage

The dosage for Maca root depends on what you are using it to treat. However, the various dosages include:

1. FOR INFERTILITY: to improve your fertility by increasing your semen and sperm count, take Maca root twice pay day for 4 month

2. FOR BOOSTING OF LIBIDO AND TREATMENT OF ERECTILE DYSFUNCTION: to enhance your libido and erection, take Maca root twice per day for 12days.

3. FOR ANXIETY AND DEPRESSION: to relief anxiety and depression, take Maca root twice per day for 10days

4. FOR BOOSTING OF IMMUNE SYSTEM, ENERGY AND STAMINA LEVEL AND TO

RELIEF THE SYMPTOMS OF MANOPAUSE:

take Maca root, twice per day for 2weeks

The Preparation of Maca Root

To prepare Maca root, kindly take the steps below:

1. Harvest some Maca root, wash it and dry it. Once it is dry, pound or chops it into smaller pieces.
2. Measure 1teaspoon and pour it into your ceramic pot with 8ounce of water and boil it for 10-15 minute.
3. Step it down and strain it.

Alternatively, measure 1tablespoon of Maca root powder if you buy it online and add it to any of your choice smoothie or juice twice per day.

Ginkgo Biloba

Ginkgo Biloba is an herbal plant that has been used by the Chinese for more than 200million years ago. I recommended this plant as part of my secrets herbs for erectile dysfunctions because, this herbs is very effective for the treatment of most of the physiological causes of erectile dysfunctions. However, because of the compound and nutrients that Ginkgo Biloba contains, research has it that tea made with the leaves of this herb is very potent in treating of anxiety, Alzheimer disease (dementia), stroke, high blood pressure, depression, multiple sclerosis etc. Don't forget that all these diseases are causes of erectile dysfunctions and this herb will help to eliminate erectile dysfunctions from it root-caused.

Precaution and Side Effects of Consuming Ginkgo Biloba

Tea made with the leaves of Ginkgo Biloba is likely safe but if it is taken in excess (overdose), you might suffer from minor side effects like: dizziness, forceful heartbeat, stomach upset and headache.

Ginkgo Biloba Dosage

The dosage for Ginkgo Biloba depends on what you are using it to treat. However, the various dosages include:

1. FOR THE TREATMENT OF DEPRESSION, ANXIETY, HIGH BLOOD PRESSURE AND BLOOD CLOT, take Ginkgo Biloba three times per day for 4 weeks (1 month)

2. FOR STROKE, take Ginkgo Biloba, 3times daily

for 14-30days

3. FOR ALZHEIMER DISEASE (DEMENTIA) AND MULTIPLE SCLEROSIS take Ginkgo Biloba three times per day for 12month.

The Preparation of Ginkgo Biloba:

For the preparation of Ginkgo Biloba, you will need to harvest some fresh leaves of Ginkgo Biloba, wash it and dry it. Once it is dried, chop it into smaller pieces and follow the under-listed steps:

1. Boil 8ounce of water and turn off the fire and measure 2teaspoon of the chopped or pounded leaves and pour it into the boiled water.
2. Allow it to steam for 5-10 minutes and strain it using a strainer or filter.

3. You are done.

Irish Sea Moss

Irish Sea Moss is also known as Sea Moss. It is a red alga that people have used it long before now for food but today it is used for the treatment of various health disorders. Because of how rich this herb is with over 92 mineral that the human body needs out of the 102, I strongly recommend this herb for the treatment of erectile dysfunctions, calming and boosting of the immune system, enrich overall mood, speed up healing, boost energy and stamina level and also, reliefs; arthritis, pain and swelling of the joint cause by inflammation, combat different types of infections etc.

The Precaution and Side Effects Of Consuming Irish Sea Moss

Irish Sea Moss is likely safe if consume in an average dosage but if consume in overdose, there is tendency of some mild side effects like

1. Burning sensation or itching of the mouth

2. Spew out or vomiting

3. Stomach upset or irritation

4. Nausea.

The Dosage Of Irish Sea Moss

The dosage of Irish Sea Moss is generic. All you have to do is to consume Irish Seas moss once per day for 2 weeks upward. (Preferably in the morning)

Preparation of Irish Sea Moss

To prepare Irish Sea Moss tea, take the under-listed steps:

1. Get either the gel or powdery form of Irish Sea Moss.

2. Boil 8ounce of water in a ceramic pot and turn the water into your tea cup/mug

3. Pour into the boiled water, 1 tablespoon of Irish Sea Moss gel or the powdery form depending on the one you have.

4. Cover the tea cup/mug and allow it to steep for 10-15minutes to dissolve completely.

5. You are done. You can now enjoy your warm tea made with Irish Sea Moss.

Panax Ginseng

Panax Ginseng is an herbal plant from northeastern China,

Siberia and Korea. I included this herb because of its potency to treat physiological causes of erectile dysfunctions such as; boosting of the brain functionality, treatment of multiple sclerosis, alzheimer disease, heart failure, diabetes, high blood pressure etc. This herb is also very effective for the treatment of erectile dysfunctions such as; boosting of libido by increasing response to sexual stimuli, prevent premature ejaculation (early orgasm), enhance athletic performance and boost energy and stamina level and a lots more.

The Precautions and Side Effects of Consuming Panax Ginseng

This herb is likely safe when consumed for the period of 6 month. Anything more than 6 month, can lead to some side effect like:

1. Insomnia,

2. Increase heart rate

3. Loss of appetite

4. Low/high blood pressure

5. Itching

6. Mood swing etc.

Therefore, this herb should not be used for more than 4month.

Dosage of Panax Ginseng

FOR THE PREVENTION OF PREMATURE EJACULATION, HEART FAILURE, DIABETES, take this herb 3times daily for 16weeks.

FOR ALZHEIMER DISEASE (DEMENTIA) AND

MULTIPLE SCLEROSIS, take Panax Ginseng 3 times daily for 12weeks

FOR HIPERTENSION, ANXIETY AND BOOSTING OF LIBIDO, take Panax Ginseng 3times per day for 8weeks

The Preparation of Panax Ginseng

Harvest some fresh root of Panax Ginseng, wash it and dried it. Pound it or chop it into smaller pieces and the steps below:

1. Measure 8-10 ounce of water and pour it into your ceramic pot and measure 2teaspoon of the chopped Panax Ginseng and add it to the water.
2. Boil the mixture for 15 minute. Once it is boiled, step it down for 5 minute and strain it using a strainer.

Yohimbe

Yohimbe is an evergreen herbal tree in which tea made with the bark of this herbal evergreen tree contains yohimbine chemicals that helps to counteract the side effects of almost all depression medication. That's not all as it also helps to boost sexual urge, treat and prevent sexual problems, obesity, high blood pressure, enrich mood, relief anxiety and depression, boost energy and stamina level and a lots more.

The Precautions and Side Effects of Consuming Yohimbe

If you consume yohimbe in a moderate amount or as tea, it side effect is almost impossible for a short period of time but if you consume it for a very long period of time (6month) and above in high dose, there are some severe side effects like:

1. Heart attack or rapid heartbeat
2. Seizure and
3. Kidney failure.

However, it has some minor side effect which includes:

1. Stomach irritation
2. Excitation
3. Anxiety
4. Tremor
5. Dizziness
6. High blood pressure
7. Sleep problems
8. Sinus pain
9. Headache
10. Drooling

11. Nausea

12. Vomiting

13. Frequent urination

14. Irritability and

15. Rash.

However, to prevent and avoid all the above side effects, only use the tea of this herb and don't use it for more than 3 month.

The Dosage of Yohimbe

FOR BOOSTING OF LIBIDO, ENEGY AND STAMINA LEVEL, take Yohimbe 3 times per day for 21days

FOR DEPRESSION, ANXIETY AND MOOD SWING, take Yohimbe 3 times per day for 10days.

FOR SEXUAL PROBLEMS, OBESITY, HIGH BLOOD

PRESSURE, take Yohimbe 3 times per day for 4weeks.

The Preparation Of Yohimbe

Harvest some barks of Yohimbe, chops or pound it into smaller pieces and dry it or you can make an order online. Once you have it, you can take the steps below:

1. Measure 8ounce of water and 1-1½ teaspoon of the chopped or pounded Yohimbe and pour it into your ceramic pot and boil it for 10-15minute.

2. Step it down and strain it using a strainer or filter.

CHAPTER FOUR
The Natural Remedy To Screw Your Woman Like A Porn Star!
Steps On How To Treat And Prevent ED Permanently

The steps to treat and prevent ED permanently include:

1. Eat only fruits, smoothies, hand-made juice and raw veggies for a period of 1week. Please take this exercise serious as you will have to purge your entire body system of toxic substances from your body system through intra-cellular cleansing.

2. Ensure you do penis stretching exercise every morning and evening for at least five minute for 21 days.

3. Avoid eating fries and using of microwaves.

4. Take your herbs for a period of 21 day (3weeks).

5. Avoid smoking and drinking of alcohol of any sort

and type.

6. Avoid man-made/canned or plastic food except for Brazil nut and hazelnut milk.

7. Avoid flaxseed and soy because of the amount of estrogen that they both contain.

8. Avoid eating meat and dietary product.

Fruits And Veggies That Helps To Enhance Blood Flow To The Penis

There are fruits and veggies that you are advice to eat because of their potency to increase blood flow to the penis and treat and prevent ED. These fruits and veggies are:

1. List Of Vegetable:
    i. Watermelon: it helps to relax the blood vessel and promote blood circulation to your penis

and also boost the rate of testosterone production. This is possible because of the compounds (lycopene and L-citrulline) that it contains.

ii. Pink grapefruits: just like watermelon, it has lycopene which helps in enhancing blood circulation to your penis.

iii. Apple: because of flavones, flavanones and anthocyanins that apple contains, its regarded as a magical herbs for people with erectile dysfunction.

iv. Banana: banana contains potassium which helps in regulating your body's sodium level and boost blood circulation to your penis.

v. Avocado: it contains zinc and Vitamin-E which makes it to lower LDL, promote blood vessel functions which include erection and enhance healthy and quality sperm with increased in testosterone level.

vi. Carrots: it contains carotenoids chemicals which is very effective in improving of sperm count, it quality and motility.

vii. Blueberries: it helps to protect penis tissues and lower chances of heart disease because of the compounds (anthocyanin's and antioxidants) that it contains.

viii. Cherries: Cherries contains anthocyanins which makes it effective in protecting the arteries wall and keeping the arteries in good health, improve blood circulation, combats free radicals etc.

ix. Peaches: same as cherries.

x. Nectarines: same as cherries.

2. List Of Nuts:

   i. Pistachio: because of the protein that pistachios contains like 'Arginine' research has it that, eating of this nut for 3 weeks helps to improve men with erectile dysfunction conditions. Pistachio is very effective for the boosting of sexual urge (libido), relaxing of the blood vessel and enhancing of good blood circulation.

   ii. Walnuts: this contains chemicals like arginine and amino acid and Vitamin-E, fiber and folic acid which helps to enhance sperm counts and motility, boost testosterone level and libido.

3. List Of Vegetables:

   i. Spinach: helps to boost testosterone level

because of the chemical (folate) that it contains

ii. Kale: just like spinach

iii. Chili peppers: because of the chemical 'capsaicin' that chili peppers contains, research has it that, the chemical helps to trigger the release of endorphins which in turns, help boost and rev up libido and promote healthy testosterone level.

iv. Tomatoes: it contains lycopene which is very effective for the treatment and prevention of prostate cancer, enhance the quality of sperm, it count and motility.

v. Garlic and onions: these vegetables contain allicin which is very effective in increasing the blood flow to the penis which in turn leads to an improved erection.

vi. Cabbage: cabbage is very rich with various

nutrients and compound like: Vitamin-C, iron, folate, beta-carotene, potassium, glucosinolate, phosphorus, magnesium, calcium, copper etc.

Because of all these compounds, cabbage is regarded as natural Viagra.

Steps on How To Takes Your Herbs and Fruit.

This routine is supposed to be for 21days. However, I will walk you through a week program and you will use the one week to design the other 2weeks programs. Please note that in this first 7days (1week), you will undergo a fast to cleanse your entire body system through an intra-cellular cleansing.

Day One

In the morning:

Start each of your days with a cup of coffee. Coffee helps in treating and preventing of erectile dysfunctions because of the caffeine that it contains. After taking your coffee, steps it down with a cup of Irish Sea Moss. (Check chapter three to see how you can prepare Irish Sea Moss tea).

Ensure you do the penis exercise and take a cup of warm tea made with Ginkgo Biloba (Check the steps on how to prepare Ginkgo Biloba tea in chapter three) before leaving for work.

By 10: am, take a cup of herbal tea made with Yohimbe, Maca root and Panax Ginseng.

By Noon:

By noon, snacks on apple, banana and cucumber and step it down with a cup of herbal tea made with Ginkgo Biloba. Ensure you consume lots of water. (Preferably, spring water)

In The Evening:

Break your fast with a delicious green smoothie made with green apple and cucumber.

To prepare green smoothie with green apple and cucumber, you will need the following ingredients:

1. 2 handful of washed and diced cabbage.
2. 1 cored and diced pieces of green apple.
3. 1/2 chopped cucumber.
4. 3-5 pieces of dates.

Remove the seeds of the dates and add the diced salad and little water into your blender and blend it until it is smooth.

Add the other ingredients and blend it until it is completely smooth.

After taking your smoothie, step it down with a cup of herbal tea made with Yohimbe, Maca root and Panax Ginseng.

Do your penis stretching exercise and after the exercise, take a cup of warm tea made with Ginkgo Biloba leafs.

Please note that you need to consume lots of water (spring water)

Day 2:

In The Morning:

Just like the 1st day, start your day with a cup of coffee and step it down with a cup of Irish Sea Moss.

After that, do the penis stretching exercise and take a cup of warm ginkgo Biloba tea before taking off for work.

By 10: am, take a cup of herbal tea made with Yohimbe, Maca root and Panax Ginseng.

By Noon:

By noon, snack on pistachio, peaches and watermelon and step it down with a tea made with Ginkgo Biloba

Please note that water is a key to flushing out all the toxic in your body system during this first week of intra-cellular cleansing.

In The Evening

End you day with a delicious smoothie made with apple, banana and watermelon. To make this smoothie, you will need the following:

1. A handful of kale
2. 1-2 bananas.

3. 1/6 of a medium size watermelon (sliced).

4. 1 cored apple.

5. Handful of walnuts.

Wash all the ingredients, peel the watermelon and leave the seed. Peel the bananas and remove the seed of the apple.

Chop all the ingredients into smaller pieces and pour it into your blender and blend it until it is completely smooth.

After drinking your smoothie, step it down with a cup of herbal tea made with Yohimbe, Maca root and Panax Ginseng.

Do your penis stretching exercise and take your herbal tea made with Ginkgo Biloba leafs.

Day 3

Just like every other day, the routine is the same but the snacks and smoothies are different.

Follow the steps in either day one or two.

By Noon, snacks on: Avocado, blueberries, pistachio, banana and carrots.

In The Evening:

The smoothie will be made with blueberries and avocado. To make this delicious smoothie, you will need the following ingredients:

1. Handful of washed spinach
2. ½ peeled, pitted and diced avocado
3. 1 Cup of blueberries
4. 1/2 cup of hazel or brazil nut milk

Pour all your ingredients into your blender and blend it

until it is completely smooth.

Day 4:

Take the same steps as the steps in day 1 or 2.

Ensure you do your penis stretching exercise, and drink lots of water.

By Noon:

Snacks on some fruits like: watermelon, banana and apple. You can also soak 2-4 walnut pieces that you will snacks on the fifth day.

In The Evening:

End your day with a delicious smoothie made with banana, carrots and apple. To make this smoothie, you will need the following ingredients:

1. Handful of washed and diced cabbage

2. 2 chopped carrots.

3. 2 ripe peeled banana.

4. 1 slice cored apple.

5. ½ cup of almond or Brazil nut milk.

Pour all the ingredients into your blender and blend it until it smooth.

Please note that, your penis stretching exercise is very important morning and evening and lots of water.

Day 5

In The Morning:

Congrats for making it this far.

The coffee and herbal teas consumption remain the same throughout the 21days program.

By Noon:

Snack on some of the fruits that help to enhance blood flows to the penis together with the walnut that you soak yesterday.

In The Evening:

End your day with green smoothie made with avocado, blueberries and banana. To make this smoothie, you will need the following ingredients:

1. ½ peel, pitted and diced avocado
2. 1 chop, peel ripe banana
3. Handful of kale
4. ½ cup of brazil nut or hazelnut milk

Wash the kale and add it to your blender and pour the milk and blend it until it is smooth.

Add the other ingredients and blend it until it is completely smooth.

Enjoy your smoothies and step it down as usual with the needed herbs.

Day 6:

In The Morning:

Today, you must have started feeling a brown new you. Though the fasting process is not easy, but we need to pay a price for everything.

Start your day as usual with a cup of coffee and make a delicious purple smoothie with cabbage, blueberries, strawberries, banana and cherry. To make this amazing smoothie, you will need the following ingredients:

1. ¼ - ½ purple cabbage (medium size)

2. 1 ripe, peel banana

3. Handful of strawberries

4. Handful of blueberries

5. Handful of cherries

6. ½ cup of Brazil nut or hazelnut milk.

Add all the ingredients together and blend it until it is completely smooth.

Ensure you do your penis exercise; take your herbal tea and lots of water.

Please note that, everything concerning the coffee and herbal teas remain the same.

By Noon:

Snacks on some fruits that help to enhance blood flow to the penis.

In The Evening:

End your day with a delicious strawberries salad made with spinach, berries and walnuts.

To make this delicious strawberry salad, you will need the following ingredients:

1. 2 handful of spinach
2. Handful of strawberries, blueberries and raspberries each.
3. Handful of toasted walnuts
4. 1 onion
5. Sea salt to taste

To prepare this salad, you will have to chop the toasted walnut into smaller pieces.

Get a bowl, wash the spinach and pour it into the bowl. Dice your onion and spray it un-top of the washed spinach.

Slice your berries and add them to the spinach.

Spray the chopped walnuts and a little sea salt to taste.

Toast it to your liking and serve.

Please note that your herbal teas and penis stretching exercise should be done as usual

Day 7:

In The Morning:

Congrats for making it to the last day of your fast.

Today just like every other day, start your day with a cup of coffee, accompanied with your herbal tea made with Irish Sea Moss.

Do your penis stretching exercise and take another cup of herbal tea made with Ginkgo Biloba leafs before leaving for work.

As usual, by 10: am, take another cup of herbal tea made with Yohimbe, Maca root and Panax Ginseng.

By Noon:

Enjoy a delicious lunch made with cabbage. To make this delicious cabbage salad, you will need the following ingredients:

1. ½ ball of medium cabbage
2. 2-3 pieces of tomatoes
3. 1 smash avocado
4. ½ medium size cucumber
5. ½ key lime
6. Sea salt to taste
7. 1-2 chili pepper
8. 1 onion

Slice and wash your cabbage and sieve the water from the cabbage and pour it into a bowl.

Slice the onion, tomatoes, chili pepper and cucumber and spray all on the cabbage.

Get another bowl, remove the seed of the avocado and remove the flesh.

Juice the key lime into the avocado and whisk it.

Turn the whisk avocado and the key lime into the salad and stir it.

Add the sea salt and stir it to taste.

After eating your lunch, steps it down with a cup of herbal tea made with Ginkgo Biloba leafs.

Please note that you need to drink lots of water.

In The Evening:

End your fast with any of your favorite's meal that you missed a lot for these periods of your fast. However, note that, you don't have to go back to eating fries, diary product, canned food etc.

After your dinner, steps it down with a cup of herbal tea made with Yohimbe, Maca root and Panax Ginseng.

Before you take off for bed, take another herbal tea made with Gingko Biloba leaves.

For the next 14 days, you will take these herbal teas as usual and the penis stretching exercise too.

Before the end of the first 7 days, you will discover a drastic change in your life.

By the end of this exercise, you will see a brand new you with a bigger, thicker, harder and long lasting erection. Not only that, you will experience a super you with hyper energy, free from any erectile dysfunction and a massive boost in your sex life.

How To Make Herbal Tea With Yohimbe, Maca Root And Panax Ginseng Combine?

To make herbal tea with Yohimbe, Maca Root and Panax Ginseng combine, take the steps bellow:

1. Measure 8-10ounce of water and 1½ teaspoon of Yohimbe chopped bark, 1teaspoon of chopped or pounded Maca root and 2teaspoon of Panax Ginseng chopped root and pour the mixture into your ceramic pot.
2. Boil the mixture for 10-15 minutes.
3. Step it down and strain it using a strainer
4. You are done and can now enjoy your herbal tea made with Yohimbe, Maca root and Panax ginseng.

How to Stretch Penis (Penis Stretching Exercise)?

To stretch your penis, use your hand to massage your penis tissue along the length. The more you stretch it, the more your penis tissues will have some micro tear which will keep making it longer and bigger. To stretch your penis, take the steps bellow:

i. Use your hand to grasp the head of your penis.

ii. Pull it upward for some seconds.

iii. Press the base of your penis and hold it for some seconds.

iv. Pull your penis upward to the left and apply pressure to the right side of the base of your penis.

v. Repeat the same process but this time, you should pull it upward to the right and apply pressure to the left side of the penis.

vi. Do this exercise morning and evening for at least 2minutes throughout the 21 days program.

Best of luck in your new sex life and thank you for journey with me into the world of pleasurable, healthy and happy sex life!

About The Book

This book was written by Clement Jacob as a guide to help both; young and old who are suffering from one form of erectile dysfunction or the other that desire a permanent cure.

According to the author, this book is key to every man from the age of 50 and above and young men as well who are finding it difficult to get and sustain erection for sexual intercourse, men who have lost their self-esteem because they have stop being the men they use to be in the bedroom, men with small penis, wen who are suffering from swing mood, low libido, premature ejaculation, low sperm count, lack enough energy and stamina to screw their woman like a porn star and anything that is related to erectile dysfunctions.

You don't want to miss this!!!

Printed in the USA
CPSIA information can be obtained
at www.ICGtesting.com
LVHW010957051023
760229LV00009B/175